PREGNANT & GOING STRONG

Exercise and Activities Guide for all 3 Trimesters.

By

CYNTHIA LEONARD

TABLE OF CONTENTS

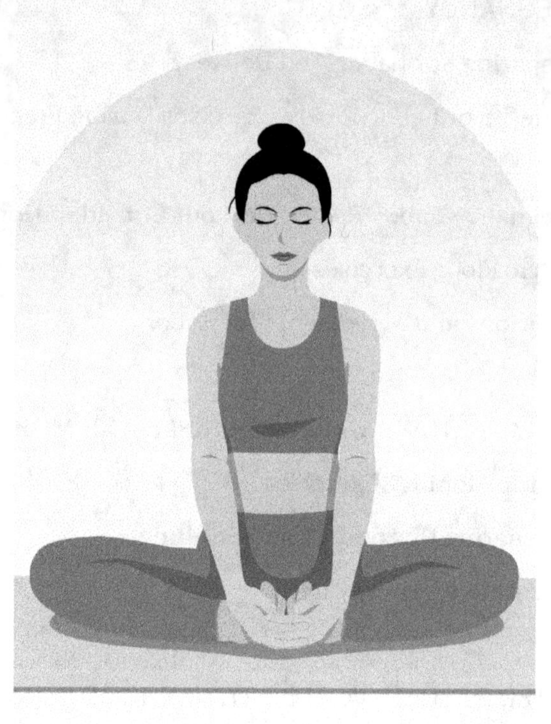

INTRODUCTION: EMBRACING PREGNANCY FITNESS

The Importance Of Staying Active During Pregnancy

Pregnancy exercise is important for the health of both the mother and the unborn child. While it's necessary to speak with your doctor before beginning any fitness programme while pregnant, remaining active within the advised parameters may have a number of advantages.

The following are some main reasons for why exercising when pregnant is crucial:

Improved Physical Health: Pregnancy-related physical exercise may help control weight gain, boost cardiovascular fitness and improve muscular tone and strength. This may promote a healthy pregnancy and make the postpartum recovery process simpler.

Exercise is known to **Produce Endorphins**, the *"feel-good"* chemicals, which may help manage mood swings, tension and anxiety associated with pregnancy. Both the mother and the growing child benefit from maintaining a cheerful outlook.

Reduction in the risk of Gestational Diabetes: Gestational diabetes may cause issues for both the mother and the unborn child. By maintaining an active lifestyle, blood sugar levels can be controlled.

Improved Sleep: Regular exercise may help with improved sleep, which is often disturbed during pregnancy owing to hormonal changes, pain and worry. For the mother's general health and the foetus's proper growth, a mother must get enough rest.

Easier Labour and Delivery: Regular exercise may help to build the muscles required for labour and delivery, which may ease the process of giving birth. Additionally, maintaining an active lifestyle helps increase stamina, which is advantageous throughout the strenuous labour and delivery process.

Improved Circulation: Due to increased strain on the blood vessels during pregnancy, edema and the chance of developing varicose veins are both enhanced. Regular exercise may enhance circulation, lowering the risk of these problems and enhancing cardiovascular health in general.

Faster Postpartum Recovery: Pregnant women who maintain their level of activity after giving birth often recover more quickly. Regaining fitness levels from before pregnancy more quickly may be facilitated by maintaining muscular strength and endurance.

Expectant women should be careful and refrain from potentially hazardous activities. In order to identify the right amount of physical activity depending on their particular health, any existing problems and the stage of pregnancy, they should speak with their doctor.

While pregnant, safety should always come first while exercising in any manner.

Setting Realistic Fitness Goals

Maintaining a woman's health during pregnancy is important and setting reasonable exercise goals should prioritise the well-being of both the mother and the unborn child.

Before starting any exercise program, consult with a healthcare professional for personalised advice. Focus on maintaining general well-being by choosing low-impact exercises like walking, swimming, stationary cycling and prenatal yoga.

Set reasonable goals, aiming for a fair level of fitness and promoting a safe pregnancy. Pay attention to your body's cues and stop exercising if you experience discomfort, lightheadedness or pain. Adjust your training plan as needed.

Keep well-hydrated and well-fed to support increased nutritional requirements during pregnancy. Focus on pelvic floor exercises, such as Kegels, to promote pelvic floor health.

Maintain good posture during pregnancy and after delivery by including posture-enhancing exercises like mild strength training or prenatal Pilates.

Incorporate relaxation methods like prenatal massage, deep breathing exercises or pregnancy meditation to manage stress, improve sleep quality and enhance overall wellbeing. Be adaptable with your training regimen as physical stamina and energy levels may change throughout pregnancy.

By setting reasonable and pregnancy-specific exercise objectives, you can ensure that you are taking care of both your personal health and the health of your growing baby.

Safety Precautions And Guidelines

To protect the safety of both the mother and the growing baby, it is essential to approach fitness during pregnancy with prudence and adhere to particular rules.

Here are some recommendations for safety measures:

Speak with your Doctor: Before beginning any fitness programme, speak with your doctor or obstetrician to make sure the activities you choose are healthy for both you and your unborn child. Based on your medical history and the particular needs of your pregnancy, they may provide tailored advice.

Exercises with Minimal Impact: Choose exercises with low impact that are soft on the joints and don't increase your chance of falling or being hurt. Prenatal yoga, swimming, stationary cycling and walking are often seen as safe activities.

Avoid High-Risk activities: Refrain from engaging in activities that increase your chance of falling or suffering abdominal injuries, such as contact sports, strenuous racquet sports, downhill skiing and impact-heavy activities.

Monitor your Heart Rate: keep an eye on your heart rate and try to maintain it within a healthy range when exercising. Always strive to keep your intensity at a level where you can easily carry on a conversation. While exercising, avoid being out of breath or worn out.

Stay Hydrated: Drink plenty of water before, during, and after exercise to avoid being dehydrated, particularly if you're doing vigorous activities that cause you to perspire.

Be Mindful of your Body: While exercising, be aware of any discomfort, pain, dizziness or shortness of breath. Stop right once and talk to your doctor if you encounter any of these signs.

Change your Exercise Regimen: As your pregnancy goes on, you may need to make some adjustments. Adjust your workouts to your changing body by adding more support, adjusting the range of motion and staying away from activities that put undue stress on your abs.

Avoid Lying flat on your Back: Exercises that require you to rest flat on your back for a lengthy amount of time should be avoided after the first trimester because they may put pressure on a major vein and may limit blood supply to the uterus.

Practise proper Nutrition: Ensure appropriate nutrition by eating a balanced diet that gives you and your baby the nutrients you need. The growth of the foetus and your energy levels are both supported by proper eating.

Prioritise Rest and Recovery: Give rest and recuperation first priority by giving yourself plenty of time in between workouts. Pay attention to your body's cues and refrain from overdoing it.

CHAPTER 1: FIRST TRIMESTER

Exercises And Activities For The Early Stages Of Pregnancy

Prioritising activities that advance the health and wellbeing of the mother and the growing foetus throughout the early stages of pregnancy is crucial. Maintaining an active lifestyle may aid with stress management, good weight maintenance and even preparing the body for the physical demands of labour.

However, it's important to speak with a doctor before beginning a new fitness programme while pregnant. During the first trimester of pregnancy, it's typically advised to do the following safe workouts and activities:

Walking: Pregnant women may typically safely engage in this low-impact cardiovascular activity. It helps to maintain a healthy weight, enhance overall mood and energy levels, and improve circulation.

Swimming is a great exercise for expecting mothers. It offers a full-body exercise without stressing the tummy and is easy on the joints. It is a great workout for pregnant women since the water helps to support the weight of the expanding abdomen.

Prenatal Yoga: Prenatal yoga is especially designed to assist expecting moms strengthen their muscles, increase their flexibility and practise breathing methods that may be helpful during labour. It also emphasises relaxation and stress reduction, which may be especially advantageous during pregnancy.

Pilates: Modified Pilates exercises may aid with improving core strength, stability, and flexibility, which can be helpful during pregnancy and labour. However, it's crucial to engage with a trained pregnant Pilates teacher who can show you movements that are secure for pregnancy.

Cycling Stationary: Another low-impact activity that might assist preserve cardiovascular health during pregnancy is stationary cycling. Because it doesn't place strain on the joints and is simple to modify to your comfort level, it is typically safe.

Low-Impact Aerobics: Attending low-impact aerobics sessions designed specifically for pregnant women may help preserve cardiovascular health, build muscle and enhance flexibility. Make sure you enrol in prenatal fitness sessions taught by qualified instructors.

Strength Training: When done under expert supervision, modest strength training activities may help maintain muscular tone and get the body ready for the physical demands of pregnancy and labour. Exercises that target large muscular groups, such as the arms, legs, back and shoulders, should be prioritised.

Always pay attention to your body's signals and stay away from any workouts that make you feel uncomfortable or uncomfortable. After the first trimester, it's important to avoid workouts that require resting flat on your back, remain hydrated and wear the right attire.

Nurturing A Strong Foundation - Gentle Stretching and Warm-Up Routines:

Warm-up exercises and gentle stretching may be quite helpful during pregnancy. They may support improved circulation, increase flexibility and lessen pain.

It is important to speak with your doctor before beginning any fitness regimen while pregnant. A basic approach to warm-up and stretching exercises is provided below:

- Before beginning any fitness programme, particularly while pregnant, speak with your medical professional. They can provide advice that is customised to your unique medical requirements and your pregnancy's stage.

- **Exercises to warm up:** Before beginning any stretching regimen, it is important to warm up. Warming up your muscles and promoting blood flow may be accomplished by engaging in a brief, mild aerobic exercise, such as walking or stationary cycling, for 5 to 10 minutes.

- Stretching your neck involves a gentle head tilt that brings your ear close to your shoulder without raising your shoulder. Hold each side for ten to fifteen seconds. Then make a gentle, circular motion with your neck.

- Stretching your arms and shoulders involves extending one across your body and applying gentle pressure with the other hand while holding the stretch for 10 to 15 seconds. Continue by using the opposite arm. By rotating your shoulders in a circular pattern, you may also do shoulder rolls.

- Stretching your chest involves placing your hands on the small of your back and gently arching your upper back. Maintain for 10 to 15 seconds.

- Gentle back stretches, like the cat-cow stretch, should be done. Get down on your hands and knees and slowly and deliberately alternately arch and round your back.

- Try modest hip-opening activities like the butterfly stretch for hip stretches. Kneel down on the floor and put your feet together with the soles touching. Holding your feet, gently raise and lower your knees.

- Stretch your legs by reaching towards your toes while standing or sitting with your back erect. Leaning against a wall and pushing one leg back while maintaining the heel on the floor are other ways to do calf stretches.

- Stretching is followed by a cool-down that involves slowing down and doing deep breathing exercises.

Drink plenty of water during your exercise to prevent dehydration and overheating and always pay attention to your body's signals. Refrain from any motions that hurt or discomfort. If you develop any strange symptoms while exercising, such as vaginal bleeding, lightheadedness or breathing difficulty, stop right away and contact your doctor.

Core Strengthening For A Stable Pelvic Floor

Exercises that strengthen your core are especially helpful for keeping a healthy pelvic floor, which helps support your expanding belly and help avoid problems like incontinence. For pregnant ladies, try these exercises for core stability:

Pelvic Tilts: Lie on your back with your legs bent and your feet flat on the ground to do pelvic tilts. Engage your core muscles as you gently tilt your pelvis forward. Hold the position for a few seconds before letting go. Several times, repeat this motion.

Pelvic Tilts

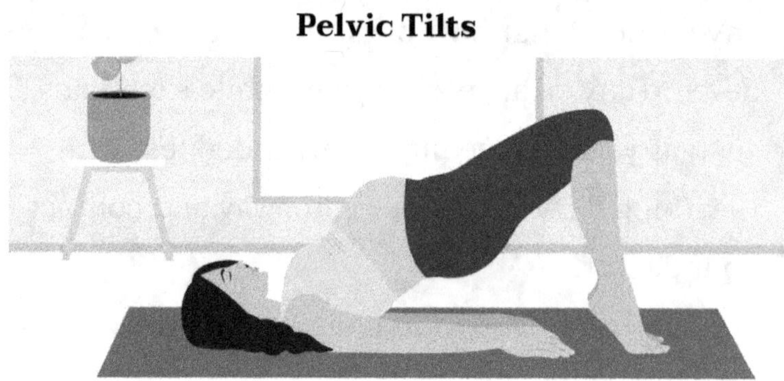

Kegel Exercises are a quick and efficient approach to build up the muscles in your pelvic floor. To do Kegels, tense the muscles in your pelvic floor as though you're attempting to block the pee from coming out. Hold for a little while, then let go. Several times during the day, repeat this.

Modified Planks: To do modified planks, go down on all fours and slowly elevate your knees off the floor while maintaining a straight back and a tight core. Before bringing your knees back down to the ground, hold this stance for a few seconds. Repeat this motion while paying attention to your core's involvement.

Side-lying Leg Lifts: Lie on your side with your legs stacked. Lift the upper leg gently while maintaining solid hips and a tight core. Reverse the process on the opposite side, lowering the leg back down. In order to maintain general core stability, the oblique muscles need to be strengthened.

Squats: Squats are great for boosting the power of your pelvic floor and other lower-body muscles. As you progressively lower yourself into a crouching posture while keeping your knees in line with your toes, start off standing with your feet hip-width apart. Repeat by rising back to the starting position.

Cat-Cow Stretch: Your spine and abdomen's strength and flexibility are both enhanced by this easy yoga position. Get down on your hands and knees and alternate between the cat posture, which involves arching your back upward, and the cow stance, which involves bringing your belly to the floor while elevating your head and tailbone.

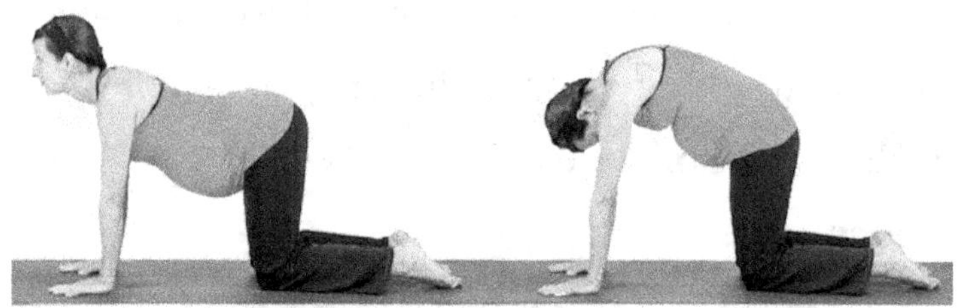

Cat-Cow Stretch

Yoga And Mindfulness For Stress Reduction

Prenatal yoga and mindfulness can be beneficial for pregnant women, as they can ease stress, promote relaxation and improve fitness alongside flexibility. To incorporate yoga and mindfulness into your prenatal exercise program, follow these guidelines:

1. Choose prenatal yoga courses designed for pregnant individuals, as they focus on secure postures and methods.

2. Focus on gentle and safe poses, avoiding positions that require prolonged back reclining or compress the abdomen. Use positions that increase flexibility and strength while ensuring the safety of both you and your infant.

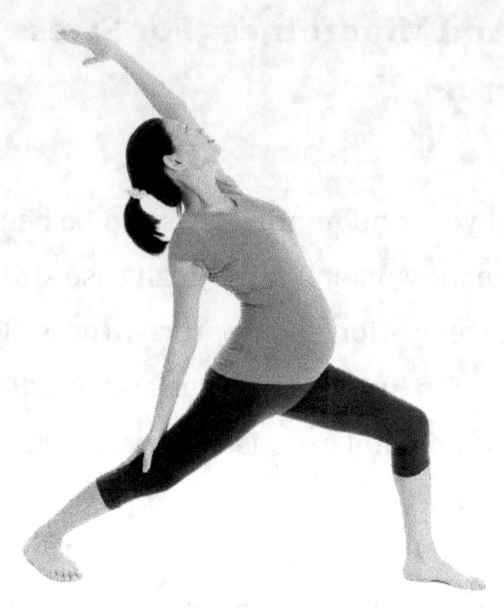

3. Practice mindfulness meditation to lower stress and support emotional wellbeing.

4. Keep hydrated and limit your activity to prevent dehydration and overheating. Avoid exercising in hot or humid conditions and ensure adequate water intake.

5. Adjust your yoga practice as needed to account for your expanding tummy and potential physical pain. Pay attention to any discomfort or warning signs and adjust as necessary.

6. Incorporate deep breathing exercises into your daily routine and yoga practice to emphasise breathing techniques.

7. Prioritise balance and stability, as your centre of gravity may fluctuate during pregnancy. Focus on postures that improve stability and balance to avoid slips and injuries.

8. Consider adding low-impact activities like walking, swimming or prenatal aerobics to your routine. Remember to pay attention to your body and adjust as necessary.

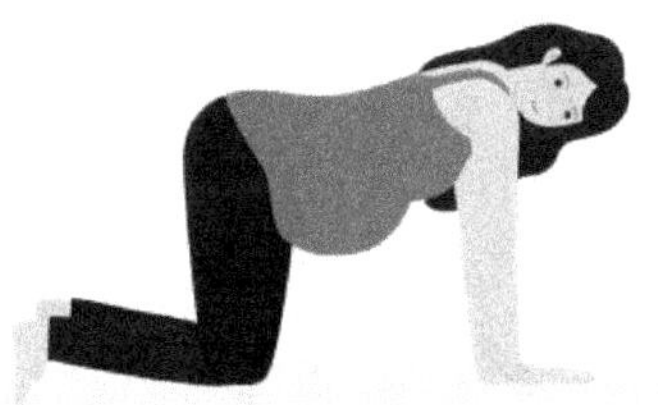

CHAPTER 2: ENERGISING YOUR FIRST TRIMESTER

Low-Impact Cardio Workouts

Since they serve to boost heart rate and circulation without placing an undue amount of stress on your joints and ligaments, low-impact cardio activities may be very helpful. Before starting any workout programme while pregnant, always check with your doctor.

Here are some low-impact cardiovascular exercises that are safe for expectant mothers:

Walking is an easy and efficient approach to increase heart rate without putting undue physical pressure on your body. You can perform it very much anyplace and you can change the tempo to suit your comfort level.

Swimming: A great low-impact workout that supports the weight of your expanding tummy is swimming. Additionally, it aids in lowering edema and joint discomfort. During pregnancy, swimming may be very calming and revitalising.

Prenatal Yoga: Prenatal yoga includes gentle postures and motions made especially for expectant mothers. Flexibility, strength and balance are all enhanced. Additionally, it encourages rest and might lessen tension.

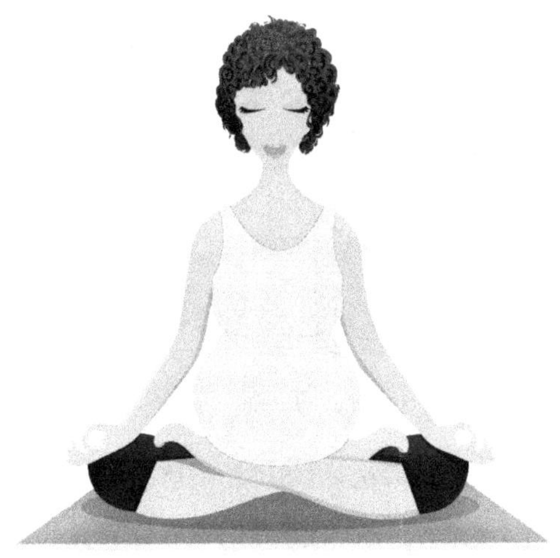

Cycling while stationary or recumbent might be a secure approach to increase heart rate without falling or losing balance. Additionally, it's an excellent technique to strengthen your legs without placing strain on your joints.

Low-impact aerobics: Attending a prenatal low-impact aerobics class or following a safe exercise regimen at home may help maintain muscle tone and enhance cardiovascular health without putting any pressure on the body.

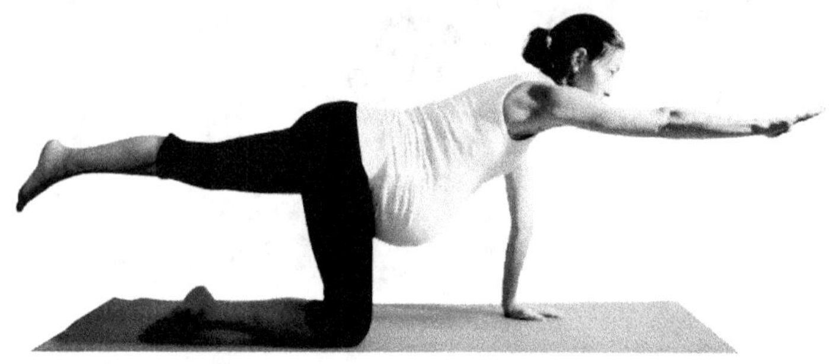

Elliptical Training: Using an elliptical machine gives your heart a decent workout while putting the least amount of stress on your joints. It helps

to preserve muscular strength and enhance
stamina.

Aerobic Exercise Modifications

Pregnancy exercise offers numerous benefits for
both the mother and the unborn child, including
improved moods, less pain and better overall
health. However, it is beneficial to adjust your
workout routine as needed to ensure the safety of
both parties. Discuss with your doctor before
starting any workout program, as they can
provide tailored guidance based on your current
health and pregnancy needs.

Incorporate low-impact workouts like walking,
swimming or stationary cycling to strengthen the
heart without straining joints.
Avoid high-impact exercises like leaping, jogging
or vigorous aerobics, as they may strain joints
and pelvic floor muscles. Reduce intensity as

needed, paying attention to your body's signals and adjusting intensity as needed.

Be sure to drink plenty of water before, during and after exercise. Start your workout with a warm-up to prepare your muscles and end with a cool-down to return your heart rate to resting levels.

Maintain a straight posture to prevent balance issues during pregnancy. Avoid workouts that require prolonged rest on your back after the first trimester, as this may strain the vena cava, the main vein supplying blood back to the heart.

Adjust exercises for comfort as your belly expands, using broader stances and providing more support to maintain balance. Also consider the weather while exercising to avoid overheating, which can harm both you and the baby.

Maintaining Balance And Coordination

For the general health of both the mother and the growing baby, it's important to maintain balance and coordination throughout pregnancy.

Regular exercise may aid with this, but it is wise to choose exercises that are safe and appropriate for your stage of pregnancy.

Following are some basic pointers and exercises to keep your balance and coordination when pregnant:

Yoga and Pilates are two workouts that may aid with coordination, flexibility and balance. Look for prenatal yoga or Pilates sessions that are especially designed with pregnant women in mind.

Walking is a low-impact activity that enhances circulation, supports a healthy body weight and helps maintain overall fitness. Additionally, it helps maintain balance and coordination.

Swimming and water aerobics are excellent choices since they provide the whole body a workout while being easy on the joints. Because of the buoyancy of the water, it is simpler to maintain balance when carrying more weight during pregnancy.

Exercises for the Pelvic Floor: Building up your pelvic floor muscles can help you maintain your balance while supporting the weight of your developing baby. Exercises for the kegel, in particular, may be advantageous.

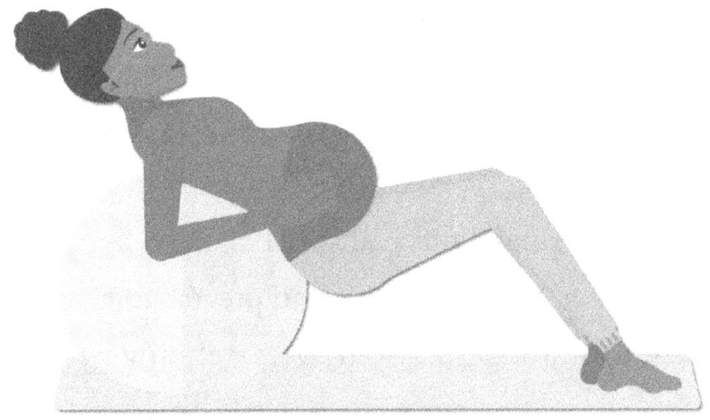

Modified Strength Training: Under the direction of a qualified trainer, choose mild strength training exercises utilising your own body weight or small weights. Exercises that enhance balance and stability should be prioritised.

Tai Chi: Tai Chi is a low-impact activity that is safe for pregnant women and may help with balance and flexibility. To find customised routines, look for pregnancy Tai Chi sessions or speak with a professional teacher.

Stretching may help you stay balanced by increasing your flexibility and preventing muscular stiffness. Avoid overextending, particularly during pregnancy when your ligaments are more pliable.

Exercises for balancing: Include easy balancing drills like heel-to-toe walking, standing on one leg with assistance and utilising a stability ball while being guided by a professional.

CHAPTER 3: CONNECTING WITH YOUR BABY

Prenatal Bonding Techniques

Expectant parents may connect with their unborn child while they are pregnant by engaging in prenatal bonding strategies. Creating a deep emotional connection with your unborn child before giving birth may be a fantastic approach to improve the parent-child bond and encourage a healthy, happy pregnancy.

The following are some prenatal bonding strategies:

Talking to Your Baby: Since a baby can hear noises made outside of the womb, chatting to your child may help you build a stronger bond. Talk to someone, sing a song or read a book out loud.

Touching and Caressing your Tummy
lightly might make you and your unborn child
feel more connected. Additionally, it may aid in
relaxation and stress relief.

Playing Music: Playing your baby's favourite or
peaceful music will help you and your baby relax.
Many parents decide to sing or play music for
their unborn children.

Meditation and Visualisation: Spend some
time in private meditation picturing a happy,
healthy future for you and your kid. This may
facilitate connection and lessen stress.

Keep a Pregnancy diary: Create a diary or
write letters to your unborn child. Keep a journal
of your ideas, emotions and experiences during

your pregnancy. When your kid is older, you can explain this to them.

Attend Prenatal Courses: Getting involved in prenatal courses or support groups may help you feel connected to other pregnant parents and foster a feeling of community. Techniques for relaxing and bonding are often covered in these seminars.

Establish a Nursery or Baby room: Setting up a nursery or baby room may increase your sense of bonding with your child. It may be lovingly and carefully decorated to provide a particular space for your child.

Observe your Baby's Motions and try to envision what they may be doing when they are still inside your womb. You could feel more attuned to the baby's presence as a result.

When you feel your baby moving within your tummy, gently place your hands on it to strengthen your bond. As a reaction, you can be kicked or nudged.

Encourage your Spouse to join you in engaging in activities that will strengthen your relationship. Additionally, your spouse may feel movements, chat, sing or read to the baby, go to prenatal visits with you and more.

Eating Well and Staying good: Maintaining a regular exercise routine and nourishing your body with a good diet will help you feel more emotionally attached to your baby and assure their wellbeing.

Foetal Photography and Ultrasound: Use ultrasound and foetal photography to establish a visual connection with your unborn child. Seeing their photograph might strengthen the feeling of closeness.

Every pregnancy is different, therefore it's important to choose bonding methods that suit you best and make you feel at ease. These activities not only help you feel closer to your unborn child but also support a happy and healthy pregnancy.

Activities For Emotional Wellbeing

During pregnancy, there are several hobbies and exercises that can improve mental wellbeing.

Yoga and meditation can help manage stress, reduce anxiety and promote relaxation. Walking can enhance cardiovascular health, lift mood and support weight maintenance.

Swimming is a low-impact workout that can relieve back pain and reduce limb edema while prenatal fitness programs can provide a caring environment and encourage regular exercise.

Attending low-impact dancing lessons can improve mood, increase energy and foster emotional health.

Tai Chi is a low-impact exercise that helps ease tension, promotes relaxation and also enhances balance, flexibility and strength. Under the supervision of a competent prenatal fitness trainer, light strength training exercises can help increase muscular strength and prepare the body for labour.

These activities can also support better mental and emotional health. By engaging in these activities, pregnant women can maintain a healthy and balanced lifestyle during their pregnancy.

Preparing for the Journey Ahead

Pregnancy is a life-changing journey for both the mother and the unborn child. Physical activity during pregnancy can enhance mood, reduce pain and facilitate labour.

To ensure safety, consult your doctor before starting any exercise program.

Low-impact workouts like prenatal yoga, swimming and strolling can strengthen muscles, increase flexibility and improve cardiovascular health without straining joints.

Pelvic floor exercises, also known as Kegels, can help strengthen pelvic floor muscles, support the baby's weight and prevent urine incontinence.

Core muscle exercises can support the back and alleviate back discomfort during pregnancy.

However, avoid conventional stomach workouts, especially after the first trimester and be mindful of posture, as your centre of gravity changes during pregnancy and focus on balance and posture-promoting workouts.

Adjust your workout regimen as needed, also be sure to consult your doctor if anything feels off.

Maintaining hydration and nutrition is important before and after exercise, as well as eating well for both you and your child. Avoid overexertion after the first trimester and avoid activities that impede blood flow to the uterus.

Deep breathing techniques can help lower tension and prepare for labour, while learning effective breathing methods can help manage pain during childbirth. Postpartum exercise should be gradually resumed, ensuring a gradual regain of stamina and strength.

CHAPTER 4: SECOND TRIMESTER

EXERCISES AND ACTIVITIES FOR THE MID-PREGNANCY MONTHS

Building Muscle Strength And Endurance

Certain workouts may not be advised depending on your health and the stage of your pregnancy. Having said that, the following general advice and exercises may assist in enhancing muscular strength and stamina throughout pregnancy:-

Consultation and Approval: Before beginning any workout programme, get your healthcare provider's advice and approval. They may provide you customised advice based on your health situation and the development of your pregnancy.

Low-Impact Aerobic Exercises: You may increase your endurance without placing too much strain on your joints by engaging in exercises like walking, swimming and stationary cycling. These workouts may enhance general stamina and cardiovascular health.

Lightweight Strength Training: Lifting light weights may assist develop muscular strength. To prevent putting any pressure on your body, it's crucial to stay away from hard lifting and concentrate instead on using smaller weights with more repetitions. Squats, lunges and modified push-ups are examples of exercises that target large muscular groups and may be useful.

Yoga during Pregnancy: Yoga during pregnancy is renowned for its capacity to enhance flexibility, balance and muscular tone. Additionally, it may aid in relaxation and stress relief. Look for prenatal yoga courses or adhere to online instructions created especially for pregnant women.

Modified Pilates exercises may help you build stronger core muscles, which can be especially useful during pregnancy and the healing process after childbirth. Again, to make sure the activities are safe for pregnant women, pick prenatal-specific programmes or routines.

Exercises for the Pelvic Floor: Also known as Kegel exercises, these exercises may help strengthen the muscles in the pelvic floor, which is advantageous both during pregnancy and after delivery. Strong pelvic floor muscles may facilitate labour and lower the risk of future incontinence.

Maintain excellent Posture: Pay attention to maintaining excellent posture during your daily activities and when you are exercising. This may lessen the likelihood of back discomfort and muscular strain.

Hydration and Rest: Drink plenty of water when working out and be sure you get enough rest. Avoid overdoing it and pay attention to your body. Stop exercising as soon as you experience any discomfort, pain or dizziness and contact your doctor.

Incorporating Resistance Training Safely

Resistance training can be beneficial for pregnant women, provided they are supervised by a healthcare physician and a qualified fitness expert. It is mandatory to consult a healthcare professional before starting any new fitness program to ensure no pregnancy-related issues or hazards are present.

Choose safe and low-impact workouts, such as squats, lunges, modified push-ups and bicep curls, also focus on appropriate form and breathing to avoid injury and strain.

Avoid overexertion and exhaustion by monitoring your heart rate and maintaining a safe heart rate of less than 140 beats per minute. Stay hydrated and well-fed, especially during pregnancy, by drinking water before, during and after exercise.

Invest in supportive clothing and shoes, such as a well-fitting sports bra and comfortable shoes, to maintain stability during exercise.

Start each workout with a light warm-up and finish with a cool-down to gradually decrease your heart rate and reduce the risk of muscular damage and pain. Be aware of any warning signals, such as vaginal bleeding, dizziness, chest discomfort, trouble breathing, headache, muscular weakness, calf pain or swelling, also reduced foetal movement, then please stop exercising immediately. If any unsettling symptoms appear, call/see your doctor.

As your pregnancy progresses, you may need to make more modifications to your workouts or move to more appropriate types of physical activity. Be willing to change your regimen to fit your body's changing needs.

Relieving Aches And Pains

Many women endure different aches and pains throughout pregnancy, including back discomfort, pelvic pain and muscle cramps. Regular exercise and physical fitness maintenance might lessen these discomforts and promote a healthy pregnancy.

During pregnancy, there are several fitness recommendations to help alleviate aches and pains. Walking is a low-impact cardiovascular workout that reduces back discomfort and aids circulation.

Swimming is another option that doesn't strain joints and can ease back discomfort and reduce edema. Yoga for expectant mothers focuses on relaxing breathing, stretching and breathing exercises to ease stress and increase flexibility.

Kegel exercises can strengthen pelvic floor muscles, preventing incontinence and preparing the body for delivery.

Pilates can help develop stronger core muscles, improve posture and reduce back discomfort. Low-impact aerobics, such as stationary cycling and elliptical machines, can help improve cardiovascular shape and build stronger legs.

Consistent stretching can increase flexibility and reduce muscle tension. Use resistance bands or light weights for strength-training activities, but avoid overexertion and heavy lifting.

Balance exercises like tai chi or modified squats can help maintain stability and avoid falls. Relaxation methods like deep breathing, mindfulness and meditation can lower stress and improve overall well being.

It's important to pay attention to your body and avoid workouts that make you uncomfortable or exhausted. Staying hydrated, dressing comfortably and warm up and cool down before and after each activity session.

CHAPTER 5: CARDIOVASCULAR HEALTH

Modified Aerobics And Cardiovascular Workouts

Pregnant women should maintain a healthy fitness routine, especially during their **Second Trimester**, to improve mood, control weight gain and prepare for labour. Recommendations for reduced aerobics and cardiovascular exercise include walking, swimming, prenatal yoga, modified aerobics, cycling while stationary, low-impact dancing classes and avoiding jarring movements are:-

- Walking is a safe, low-impact cardiovascular activity suitable for most pregnant women, with at least 30 minutes of walking per week and swimming is a great full-body exercise that enhances

strength, flexibility and cardiovascular
health.

- Prenatal yoga can help increase muscular
  tone, flexibility and balance, while also
  promoting relaxation and breathing
  exercises.

- Modified aerobics regimens should focus
  on low-impact routines, avoiding exercises
  that strain the back or abdomen. Also
  cycling while stationary is a healthy
  approach to increase heart rate without
  putting undue strain on joints.

- Participating in low-impact dancing classes
  or workouts specifically designed for
  pregnant women is also beneficial.

Be sure to listen to your body's signals and stop exercising if you experience discomfort, lightheadedness or breathing difficulties and also maintaining a balanced diet can also aid your fitness program.

After the first trimester, avoid flat-backed workouts to prevent blood circulation issues. If you have any concerns or questions about your workout regimen, consult and review with your healthcare professional.

Swimming and Water Aerobics

Pregnant women may exercise safely and effectively while swimming and doing water aerobics. They provide a variety of advantages for both physical and mental health, including stronger muscles, better cardiovascular health and general well-being.

Pregnant women must, however, get approval from their doctor before starting any new workout regimen. I've included a thorough resource with specific information on swimming and water aerobics for pregnant women below:

Pregnant Women and Swimming

Advantages of Swimming While Pregnant:

- It offers a low-impact cardiovascular exercise that enhances circulation and supports heart health.

- Water's buoyancy lessens the force on joints and provides relief from frequent pregnant aches and pains including back pain and swelling.

- Swimming contributes to overall fitness levels by assisting in the development and maintenance of muscular strength and endurance.

- It encourages calmness and stress reduction, which might be especially advantageous during pregnancy.

Safety Precautions and Measures

- A healthcare professional should always be consulted before beginning any new fitness programme, including swimming.

- Diving should be avoided by expectant mothers since it might cause a sharp drop in blood pressure.

- To avoid sliding or falling, use caution while entering and leaving the pool.

- Take frequent rests and drink plenty of
water to prevent being too hot.

Techniques for Pregnant Women Swimming

- To prevent placing too much stress on the
abdominal muscles, concentrate on using
moderate strokes like the breaststroke and
backstroke.

- To keep the body and the baby receiving a
regular supply of oxygen, use regulated
breathing methods.

- For added stability and support, use pool
accessories like kickboards or flotation
devices.

The Best Techniques for Swimming when Pregnant are:

As your pregnancy advances, start out cautiously and progressively increase the intensity and length of your swimming workouts.

Pay attention to your body and refrain from exerting yourself excessively or pushing yourself.

Wear a pregnant swimwear that supports your developing belly and is cosy and comfy.

Water Exercise for Expectant Women

Water aerobics Exercises Are Beneficial during Pregnancy:

A secure and efficient method of preserving cardiovascular health and muscular strength throughout pregnancy is water aerobics.

- Common discomforts including back pain, edema and joint stiffness are lessened by it.

- Water's cushioning properties lessen the likelihood of damage and the force on the joints.

- Without placing undue effort on the body, water resistance improves muscular tone and flexibility.

Safety Precautions and Measures:

Before beginning any water aerobics programme while pregnant, always check with your healthcare professional.

Avoid vigorous motions and overuse that might irritate or strain the abdominal muscles.

Select a trainer who is educated about safe and effective workouts for pregnant women.

Techniques for Pregnant Women Using Water Aerobics:

Put your attention on slow, controlled motions that improve your cardiovascular and muscular flexibility.

Include core-focused workouts to strengthen the muscles that support the spine and posture.

To improve muscular toning, utilise water weights or resistance gear made expressly for usage in water.

Best Practises for Pregnancy Water Aerobics

- To preserve stability and comfort in the pool, choose a supportive pregnancy swimwear and suitable water shoes.
- To avoid overheating and dehydration, stay hydrated during the exercise and take breaks as necessary.

Pay attention to your body's signals and adjust your workouts as needed to suit your changing demands throughout pregnancy.

Breathing Techniques For Stamina

Particularly during pregnancy, breathing exercises may be quite beneficial for increasing stamina and general wellbeing. Maintaining a healthy lifestyle at this period may be greatly helped by engaging in the proper workouts and fitness activities.

However, since individual circumstances might change, it is essential to speak with a healthcare provider before starting any new fitness programmes, particularly while pregnant.

An extensive guide on breathing strategies for pregnant exercise and fitness may be found here:

Diaphragmatic breathing, often known as deep breathing, is a method that includes taking a deep breath in, letting the diaphragm completely expand and then slowly expelling.

It helps to increase calm and enhance oxygen flow. To ensure that the spine stays straight, pregnant women may practise this exercise whether sitting, laying down or standing. This method aids in mental relaxation and stress reduction, which improves stamina.

Pursed Lip Breathing: Pursed lip breathing is the practice of taking slow, deep breaths through the nose while softly releasing them via pursed lips. This method may help pregnant women maintain endurance during exercise while also managing breathing during physical activity and reducing shortness of breath.

Alternate Nostril Breathing: Using the thumb and ring finger to alternately shut one nostril while breathing in and out of the other, this classic yogic breathing practice is known as alternating nostril breathing *(Nadi Shodhana)*. Nadi Shodhana promotes a regular flow of oxygen throughout the body, which balances energy, lowers anxiety and boosts endurance.

Ujjayi Breathing *(Ocean Breath)*: Ujjayi breathing is the practice of breathing in and out via the nose while slightly restricting the back of the throat. This method produces a gentle, calming sound reminiscent of ocean waves that helps pregnant women relax, expand their lung capacity and retain their stamina throughout exercises.

Belly Breathing: Breathing deeply into the abdomen, expanding the belly and ensuring that the diaphragm goes lower during inhalation are the main goals of belly breathing *(also known as abdominal or abdominal-diaphragmatic breathing)*. This method may be used by expectant women to increase oxygen intake, lower stress levels and increase endurance throughout different exercise activities.

Box Breathing *(Square Breathing)*: Box breathing entails taking a deep breath in for four counts, holding it for four counts, gently expelling for four counts and then repeating the cycle four more times. Using this method while exercising during pregnancy aids in lowering stress, enhancing focus and boosting general stamina.

It is essential to put safety and comfort first while doing any workout activities during pregnancy. Pregnant women should avoid strenuous activity, drink enough water and be aware of any pain or warning symptoms.

By combining these breathing exercises with suitable prenatal workouts like yoga, walking, swimming and low-impact aerobics, you may help keep your stamina up and promote general health while you're pregnant.

CHAPTER 6: MIND-BODY HARMONY

Prenatal Yoga And Pilates

Popular exercises that are good for pregnant women include prenatal yoga and Pilates. It is important to plan with a healthcare professional before beginning any new fitness programme while pregnant to make sure it is secure for both you and your unborn child.

Prenatal Yoga: Prenatal yoga is a kind of yoga created especially for expectant mothers. It usually focuses on relaxing movements, moderate stretching and breathing exercises that may assist with balance, flexibility, strength and stress management. Back pain, motion sickness and sleeplessness are just a few of the usual pregnant aches and pains that prenatal yoga may assist with. It may also help women get ready for labour by teaching them how to regulate their breathing and maintain their composure.

Prenatal Pilates: Specially designed for pregnant women, prenatal Pilates is a modified form of standard Pilates. It places a strong emphasis on building core stability, flexibility, and muscular tone, especially in the back, abdominal and pelvic floor muscles.

Pilates workouts for pregnant women often concentrate on enhancing posture, boosting stability and supporting the spine, which may be particularly helpful as the body changes throughout pregnancy. This kind of activity could also aid in preparing the body for labour and the healing period after childbirth.

Keeping the following in mind is crucial while doing pregnant yoga or Pilates:

- Avoid overexertion by paying attention to your body.

- Keep hydrated and stop as necessary.

- After the first trimester, stay away from workouts that require you to lie flat on your back since they might impede blood flow to the uterus.

- Select a prenatal yoga or Pilates teacher with certification who has knowledge of teaching pregnant ladies.

- Your pregnancy, any difficulties and your level of fitness should all be disclosed to the fitness trainer or your doctor.

- Keep an eye out for any warning symptoms, such as vaginal bleeding, fainting or shortness of breath and contact your doctor right once if you do.

Always put your and your child's safety first while exercising.

Meditation and Relaxation Strategies

Although it may be a joyful time for women, pregnancy can also be physically and emotionally taxing. The **Second trimester**, sometimes referred to as the **"honeymoon phase"** of pregnancy, is a wonderful time to engage in relaxation techniques like meditation to aid with stress management, enhance general wellbeing, and strengthen bonds with the developing baby.

Pregnant ladies should think about the following methods throughout their second trimester:

Deep breathing exercises should be done mindfully to enhance relaxation and lower tension. Try the 4-7-8 breathing method: take a slow, 4-second breath in, hold it for 7 seconds, and then let it out for 8 seconds.

Use guided imagery to picture a tranquil setting, such as a beach or a forest. To induce a soothing mental getaway, picture the sights, sounds and fragrances.

Prenatal Yoga: Attend a prenatal yoga session or practise at home with a teacher's assistance. Prenatal yoga encourages greater sleep and flexibility while lowering stress.

Progressive Muscle Relaxation: Start at your toes and work your way up to your head, tensing and relaxing each muscle group. This method may aid in easing bodily tension and encouraging relaxation in general.

Prenatal Massage: Take into account obtaining a prenatal massage from a licensed therapist with expertise treating pregnant clients. It may ease stress and muscular tension and enhance general wellbeing.

Strolling In Nature: Spend some time strolling around a tranquil, natural area, like a park or garden. Connect with the natural world and let the peaceful surroundings relax your body and mind.

Journaling: Keep a pregnancy journal to record your emotions, ideas and experiences. By keeping a journal, you may analyse your feelings and produce a priceless memento for later reflection.

Listening to relaxing Music: To help you relax and feel peaceful, try listening to some relaxing music. It may be very beneficial to listen to classical music, natural noises or guided meditation programmes.

Bonding with the Baby: Spend some time connecting with your infant to form a bond. Sing, read or converse with your child. Both the mother and the child may feel more connected and content as a result.

Healthy Lifestyle: Eat wholesome meals, keep hydrated and get enough sleep to maintain a healthy lifestyle. The general state of well-being during pregnancy may also be influenced by a balanced diet and consistent exercise.

Promoting Positive Body Image

Pregnant mothers' emotional and physical health are significantly influenced by their body image during pregnancy. To maintain a positive body image, it is essential to seek a professional before starting any exercise program.

Choose pregnancy-safe exercises such as walking, swimming, stationary cycling, prenatal yoga and modified Pilates.

Embrace the physical changes your body undergoes during pregnancy, acknowledging that these changes are normal and important for the infant's growth and development.

Exercises that emphasise strength and flexibility can help ease some of the usual discomforts. Mindfulness and meditation practices can also help foster a positive outlook and reduce stress.

Participate in support groups that provide assistance to expectant mothers, sharing worries and experiences with others.

Wear comfortable clothing for pregnancy exercise, enhancing comfort and promoting a positive body image.

Maintaining a balanced diet that is both nutritious for the mother and the developing foetus is mandatory to improve overall health and can affect the pregnant woman's perception of her body.

Individual self-care practices, such as prenatal massages, warm baths and leisurely walks, can help reduce stress and promote a good body image. Also celebrate the journey of pregnancy and the transformations that your body undergoes, this will give you a positive attitude towards your changing body.

A diverse approach to supporting a pregnant mother's physical and mental wellbeing while promoting a good body image is essential.

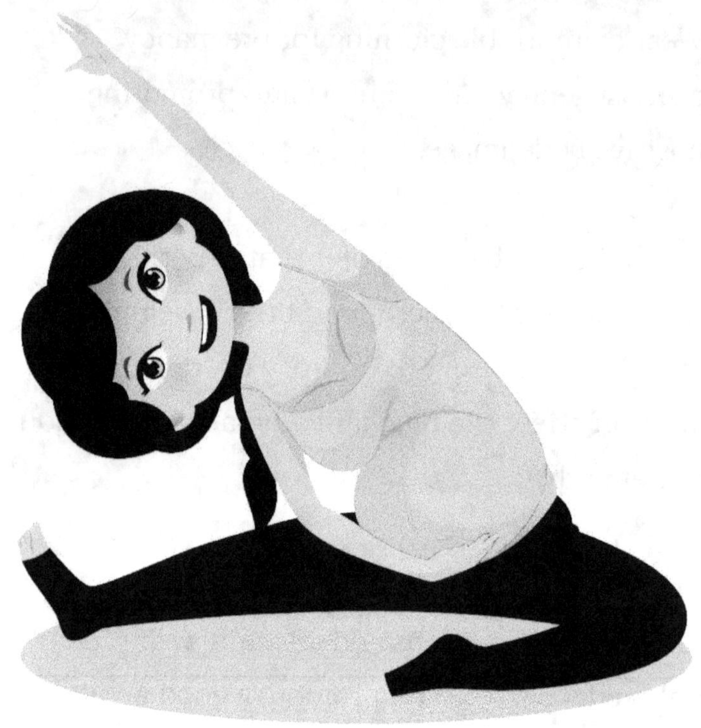

CHAPTER 7: THIRD TRIMESTER

EXERCISES AND ACTIVITIES FOR THE FINAL MONTHS OF PREGNANCY

Preparing For Labor And Delivery

Women's bodies and minds change throughout pregnancy, both physically and psychologically. Expectant moms often look for strategies to get their bodies ready for the rigours of labour since they are about to welcome a new life.

Incorporating labour-ready exercises into prenatal fitness regimens has received more attention in recent years. These specific workout plans are designed to not only support women's physical health but also provide them the stamina and fortitude to face the difficulties of delivery. Explore the significance of pregnant labour-ready workouts, stressing their advantages, suggested routines and possible pregnancy-related issues.

Benefits of Labor-Ready Exercises During Pregnancy:

Pregnancy labour-ready exercises provide a number of advantages that aid both the mother's health and the delivering process. First of all, these exercises assist in strengthening the body generally, especially the pelvic and core muscles, which are essential for labour and delivery.

Increased muscular tone may shorten labour by allowing for more efficient contractions and better placement of the baby in the delivery canal. Regular exercise may also improve a pregnant woman's general quality of life by easing typical aches and pains including back pain, swelling and exhaustion.

In addition, labour-ready exercises improve cardiovascular health, which is helpful since labour demands a lot of stamina.

Pregnant women may better handle the physical demands of delivery, such as pushing during the second stage of labour and protracted contractions by increasing their cardiovascular fitness. Also these activities may improve mental health by lowering stress and anxiety, encouraging a positive outlook and boosting self-confidence—all of which are essential components for a great delivery experience.

A. Labor-Ready Workouts:

Exercises to Get Labour Ready During Pregnancy:

Kegels: The pelvic floor muscles, which support the bladder, uterus and intestines, are strengthened by these exercises. These muscles may be made stronger to help with labour management and postpartum rehabilitation.

Squats: Squats improve balance and stability during labour by strengthening the muscles in the pelvis and legs. Additionally, they promote an open pelvis, which could make delivery simpler.

Yoga and Pilates: These exercises improve posture, flexibility and relaxation—all of which are crucial for coping with the mental and physical strains of pregnancy and labour.

Exercises that Build Cardiovascular Endurance – Walking, swimming and stationary cycling are low-impact sports that help build cardiovascular endurance, preparing expecting moms for the stamina needed during labour.

Breathing exercises: Methods like concentrated breathwork and deep breathing assist labouring women keep calm and in control while also supporting effective oxygenation for both the mother and the baby.

Pregnancy Labor-Ready Workout Considerations:

An empowering approach to prenatal fitness, pregnancy labour-ready exercises provide pregnant moms the physical and emotional fortitude required for a happy childbirth experience.

These exercises improve the general health of both the mother and the unborn child by emphasising physical strength, encouraging endurance and encouraging a positive outlook.

Labour-ready exercises may significantly contribute to the promotion of a safe and successful birthing experience when paired with adequate medical assistance and a holistic approach to prenatal care.

Pelvic Floor Exercises

Exercises for the pelvic floor are especially advised during pregnancy since they support the uterus, bladder and intestines by strengthening the supporting muscles. Having strong pelvic floor muscles may help in labour and delivery and postpartum rehabilitation.

A list of some good pelvic floor exercises to do while pregnant:

The most popular pelvic floor exercises are known as **kegels**. Follow these steps to do kegels:

- Comfortably sit, stand or lay down.

- Try to halt the flow of pee by squeezing your pelvic floor muscles.

- Hold the contraction for three to five seconds, then let it go for the same amount of time.

- 10-15 times during the day, repeat this routine.

Squats: While strengthening other muscle groups, squats may assist strengthen the pelvic floor. To safely execute squats while pregnant:

- Place your feet shoulder-width apart as you stand.

- Slowly lower your body as if you were reclining on a chair.

- Keep your knees behind your toes and your back straight.

- Return to the starting posture by standing up.

- 3 sets of 10–15 repetitions are your goal.

Pelvic Tilts: Pelvic tilts work the muscles in your lower back and abdomen, which support your pelvic floor indirectly. What to do is as follows:

- Get on your hands and knees, making sure your knees are precisely under your hips and your hands are squarely beneath your shoulders.

- Lifting your back up, gently move your belly button towards your spine.
- Hold for a little while, then let go and swing your back to the side.

- 10 to 15 times, then.

Bridge Pose: The yoga position known as bridge pose helps to relieve back pain by strengthening the pelvic floor. Take these actions:

- Your feet should be flat on the floor while you lay on your back with your knees bent.
- While maintaining your shoulders and feet firmly planted, raise your hips.
- After a little period of holding, carefully bring your hips back to the floor.

- 10 to 15 times, then.

Positions and Movements for Labor

Prenatal exercises and postures can help prepare the body for labour. Pelvic tilts increase lower back flexibility and strengthen abdominal muscles. Squats build pelvic and thigh muscles essential for labour and delivery. Kegel exercises help build pelvic floor muscles, which can be beneficial during labour and reduce postpartum incontinence.

Walking helps maintain heart health during pregnancy, while swimming strengthens muscles and enhances cardiovascular endurance. Swimming can also alleviate back discomfort and puffiness. Prenatal yoga aids in circulation, flexibility, balance, relaxation and stress reduction, which are beneficial during pregnancy and labour.

Yoga positions like the child's pose and the cat-cow stretch can soothe back discomfort and improve pelvic flexibility. Prenatal cardio workouts, such as stationary cycling or low-impact aerobics, can help maintain general fitness and heart health. However, it is important to check the appropriateness of the effort level and consult a prenatal fitness expert before starting any exercise routine.

CHAPTER 8: STAYING COMFORTABLE AND MOBILE

Gentle Mobility Exercises

The majority of pregnant women are typically regarded safe to do the following mild mobility exercises:

Pelvic Tilts: Pelvic tilts serve to build abdominal strength and increase lower back flexibility. Get on your hands and knees and slowly tilt your pelvis forward and backward to complete this exercise.

Kegel exercises: Kegel exercises serve to build up the muscles in the pelvic floor, which may support and help manage the bladder throughout pregnancy and after delivery. Simply contract your pelvic floor muscles, hold them for a few seconds and then let go to do a Kegel.

Prenatal Yoga: Prenatal yoga may aid with circulation, flexibility, balance and stress reduction while also promoting relaxation. Find a prenatal yoga class or practise prenatal yoga by watching online videos taught by a licensed teacher.

Walking: Staying active throughout pregnancy might be aided by this low-impact cardiovascular activity. To reduce your chance of falling, wear comfortable shoes and seek level surfaces.

Swimming: Because it is a low-impact sport that supports your body weight, swimming is a fantastic method to keep active throughout pregnancy. It may reduce edema and back discomfort.

Modified Squats: Squats may assist your legs become more flexible and stronger. To prevent hurting your back and knees, be careful to practise modified squats, keeping your back straight and not crouching too deeply.

Arm and shoulder circles: These may ease tension and increase flexibility in the upper body. Simply rotate your arms and shoulders clockwise and anticlockwise while standing or sitting comfortably.

Exercises that include deep breathing may help people relax and decrease tension. Inhale deeply through your nose and gently exhale through your mouth to practise deep breathing.

Alleviating Discomfort and Swelling

For many women, becoming pregnant may be a delightful and life-changing event, but it can also come with a number of discomforts and difficulties.

Following are some suggestions that may assist if you are feeling uncomfortable or swollen during pregnant:

Keep Moving: Consistent, light exercise might assist to improve circulation and minimise edema. Prenatal yoga, swimming and walking are all excellent possibilities, but before beginning any new fitness programme, check with your doctor.

Elevate Your Legs: By raising your legs, you may lessen ankle and foot edema. while you can, try to raise your legs, particularly while you're relaxing or sleeping.

Keep Hydrated: Water retention, which may cause swelling, can be avoided by drinking enough of water. To the extent that your doctor doesn't suggest differently, try to consume at least 8 to 10 glasses of water daily.

Eating a healthy diet that is balanced and rich in fruits, vegetables and whole grains will help avoid constipation and lessen edema. Reducing salt consumption may also aid in lowering water retention.

Wear Comfy Shoes: Choose supportive, comfortable footwear that gives your feet ample space. Avoid wearing high heels, which may worsen swelling and pain.

Compression clothing: Putting on a pair of compression stockings will aid your legs' circulation and minimise edema. Look for pregnancy compression socks that are made just for expectant mothers.

Rest and sleep: It's mandatory to get plenty of both throughout pregnancy. If you're uncomfortable, attempt to find a sleeping posture where your body is supported by pillows.

Massage: Light massages might aid with circulation and edema reduction. You could think about booking an appointment with a licensed prenatal massage therapist.

Cool Compresses: Using cool compresses on the affected area or bathing your feet in cool water might help ease pain and decrease swelling.

Consult Your Healthcare practitioner: If you are pregnant and suffering significant or ongoing swelling and pain, always contact your healthcare practitioner. They may provide individualised recommendations for treatments or other measures.

Maintaining Energy Levels

The health of the mother and the unborn child during pregnancy depends on the woman's ability to maintain her energy levels. To control her energy levels, focus on a well-balanced diet containing fruits, vegetables, whole grains, lean meats and healthy fats.

Eat five to six short meals daily to avoid energy slumps and maintain a steady blood sugar level. Drink plenty of water to stay hydrated and prevent fatigue-causing dehydration. Regular exercise, such as prenatal workouts or sports like swimming, walking or yoga, can improve energy levels and overall well being.

Ensure adequate rest and sleep by aiming for seven to nine hours of good sleep each night throughout pregnancy.

Control stress through relaxation techniques like pregnant yoga, meditation or deep breathing. Be sure to discuss taking prenatal vitamins and supplements with your doctor to prevent nutritional deficiencies that may lead to exhaustion. Also limit caffeine consumption to avoid energy collapses and impact the unborn child.

Observe your body when you feel fatigued and pay attention to your body's cues. If you feel lethargic or worried about your energy levels during pregnancy, consult your doctor or a prenatal counsellor for guidance and assistance.

CHAPTER 9: THE ROAD TO MOTHERHOOD

Preparing For The Postpartum Period

For the sake of both the mother and the baby's health, it is important to prepare for the postpartum period. This time frame, sometimes known as the **"fourth trimester,"** may be emotionally and physically taxing.

The following actions will assist you in getting ready for the postpartum period:

Assemble a System of Support:
Contact your friends and relatives to see if they can provide you any emotional or practical help at this time. It's essential to have individuals you can turn to for support and solace.

Make a Plan: Stock up on necessities including food, cleaning materials and baby items. This may lessen the desire to go errands in the first few weeks after giving birth.

Prepare Meals:

Consider food delivery services or prepare and freeze meals ahead of time. This guarantees that you will get wholesome meals without having to worry about cooking.

Organise Help:

Use a postpartum doula if you can, or think about hiring a nanny or babysitter to help out with childcare when necessary.

Understanding Postpartum Depression Symptoms

Know the signs of postpartum anxiety and depression and have a strategy for getting treatment if you need it. This may include

speaking with a therapist or your healthcare
practitioner.

Sleep and Rest:

The postpartum healing process requires rest.
Make an effort to sleep when the baby does, and
make sure your sleeping space is cosy.

Create Reasonable Expectations:

Recognise that the postpartum period is a time of
healing and adjustment. Do not place too much
pressure on yourself to recover right away.

Baby Necessities:

Prepare all the required baby supplies, including
diapers, clothes, a bassinet or cot, baby-safe
items and feeding apparatus.

Supplying Postpartum Care:

To help you recuperate, stock up on supplies like
sanitary pads, perineal care products and cosy
apparel.

Breastfeeding Assistance:

If you want to breastfeed, familiarise yourself with proper procedures and think about keeping a lactation consultant's contact information on hand for help.

Emotional Assistance:

During this period, be upfront with your spouse about your wants and feelings. Supporting your mental health might come mostly from your spouse.

Self-Care:

Spend some time on self-care, even if it's only for a little while. You may reenergize by taking a shower, going for a little stroll or engaging in deep breathing exercises.

Contact Siblings/Support system in advance:

If you have older kids, let them know the new baby is coming and include them in age-appropriate activities to make them feel included.

Recognise the Expectations for Recovery:
Learn about the bodily changes that may occur during postpartum recovery, such as pelvic discomfort, uterine contractions and vaginal bleeding.

Health Examinations:
To keep an eye on your physical and mental well, make an appointment for your postpartum visit with your healthcare provider.

Every woman's postpartum experience is different, so it's **OK** to ask for assistance and modify your plans as necessary. Make self-care, connecting with your child and getting help when you need it are your top priorities to make the postpartum time as easy as possible.

Building a Support System

For emotional, physical and mental health throughout pregnancy, developing a solid support network is essential. Here are some actions you can do to build a strong support system:

Support from a partner: Encourage your spouse to participate in the process. Make arrangements for the baby's arrival, talk about your thoughts and go to doctor's visits together.

Participate in the pregnancy process with your immediate and extended family. Tell them about your experiences, ask for suggestions and let them help with the baby's preparations.

Lean on close friends for support and advice when you need it most. A new viewpoint and a feeling of normality may be provided by friends in the midst of the upheavals that pregnancy brings.

Join Support Groups: Sign up for local or online pregnancy support groups. These groups provide a forum for exchanging knowledge, concerns and suggestions. In the experiences of those who are going through a similar stage, you might find comfort.

Healthcare Professionals: Build strong bonds with your medical professionals. Throughout your pregnancy, your obstetrician, midwife or doula may provide you invaluable advice and comfort if you trust them and are honest with them.

Attend prenatal seminars or courses to learn about labour, nursing and infant care. In addition to imparting useful information, these programmes provide a chance to interact with other expectant parents.

Support for your physical and emotional well-being: Think about engaging in prenatal yoga, meditation or mindfulness exercises. These pursuits may lessen your stress levels and keep your physical and mental well-being in check.

Search for local services in your area that might help expectant mothers. These can include classes on parenting, support groups for breastfeeding or counselling services specifically designed for expectant women.

Online Resources: To gain knowledge and interact with other pregnant parents, use online resources like pregnancy forums, blogs and reliable websites. These platforms may put a wealth of knowledge and assistance at your disposal.

Support from a professional: If you're having trouble coping with your emotions or have mental health issues, you may want to consider getting help from a mental health expert. They can provide you the skills you need to handle any emotional problems you could have during pregnancy, including anxiety and stress.

Celebrating Your Pregnancy Fitness Journey

Celebrating your pregnant fitness journey is a great way to appreciate the power and resilience of your body during this transforming period. It's important to respect your progress and the victories you've had both emotionally and physically.

Consider your progress by keeping a notebook or taking photographs to chronicle your pregnancy fitness experience. Create a celebration with close friends and family to discuss your struggles and express appreciation for the help you've had along the way.

Indulge yourself with a special indulgence that encourages relaxation and self-care, such as a soothing prenatal massage or a spa day. This will help you show your appreciation for your health.

Make a personal memento representing your prenatal fitness adventure by creating a pregnant fitness souvenir, such as jewellery, framed sayings or original art.

Consider creating new exercise goals that are suitable for your pregnancy stage and postpartum time, consulting with your healthcare physician or a fitness expert.

Tell others about your experiences with pregnant fitness to motivate and inspire other expectant moms on their fitness journeys. Practice expressing thankfulness for your body and the life that is developing inside you, such as mindfulness meditation, gratitude journaling or other relaxation techniques.

Celebrate your pregnancy in a way that feels meaningful and genuine to you, as every pregnancy is different. Accept the wonder of this life-changing journey and the amazing courage you have shown thus far.

CONCLUSION: A HEALTHY START TO MOTHERHOOD

The transition into motherhood is a transformative period that offers both joy and challenges. Prioritising maternal health is crucial for the welfare of both the mother and the infant, as the body undergoes various changes during and after delivery.

A supportive environment is essential for the mother to recover and enter her parental role with vigour. Postpartum health care is important for a smooth transition, promoting physical and emotional well-being through comprehensive approaches such as physical healing, emotional support and educational counselling.

The postpartum phase requires careful attention to the mother's physical rehabilitation, emphasising sleep, eating well and receiving appropriate medical treatment. Addressing post-delivery issues promptly can reduce health risks and ease the transition into the demanding role of mother.

Recognizing the emotional complexities of the postpartum period is essential, as postpartum depression and anxiety can affect mothers due to hormonal changes and the demanding duties of caring for a baby.

Providing women with educational advice on child care, nursing and self-care practices increases their confidence in carrying out their parental responsibilities. A holistic strategy that considers both the mother's and the baby's needs is essential for a healthy pregnancy and birth.

"Embrace motherhood's journey with each stride, stretch and graceful swing. Make your exercise a love symphony that shapes not just your physique but also the wonder of life within.
May each movement be a celebration of strength, resilience and the tremendous beauty of creating a new LIFE."

www.ingramcontent.com/pod-product-compliance
Lightning Source LLC
Chambersburg PA
CBHW070903260726

48661CB00004B/1578